EMS Report Writing:

A pocket reference

TODD M. STANFORD, PA, MICP

BRADY
Prentice Hall Career & Technology
Upper Saddle River, New Jersey 07458

Library of Congress Cataloging-in-Publication Data

Stanford, Todd.
    EMS report writing : a pocket reference / Todd Stanford.
      p. cm.
    ''A Brady book.''
    ISBN 0-89303-823-7
    1. Communication in emergency medicine—Handbooks, manuals, etc.
2. Medical records—Handbooks, manuals, etc. 3. Emergency medical
technicians—Handbooks, manuals, etc. I. Title.
RC86.3.S73 1992
616.02'5—dc20   91-3470
                                                CIP

Editorial/production supervision and
  interior design: **Lillian Goode**
Cover design: **Karen Marsilio**
Manufacturing buyers: **Ilene Levy/Ed O'Dougherty**
Acquisitions Editor: **Natalie Anderson**
Editorial Assistant: **Louise Fullam**

© 1992 by Prentice Hall Career & Technology
Prentice-Hall. Inc.
A Pearson Education Company
Upper Saddle River, NJ 07458

Printed in the United States of America

12

ISBN 0-89303-823-7

Prentice-Hall International (UK) Limited,London
Prentice-Hall of Australia Pty. Limited, Sydney
Prentice-Hall Canada Inc., Toronto
Prentice-Hall Hispanoamericana, S.A., Mexico
Prentice-Hall of India Private Limited, New Delhi
Prentice-Hall of Japan, Inc., Tokyo
Pearson Education Asia Pte. Ltd., Singapore
Editora Prentice-Hall do Brasil, Ltda., Rio de Janeiro

Contents

I would like to dedicate this work to the folks from whom I have learned so much: to my instructors, peers, and patients; to my family, who contributed to the realization of this goal, especially my dear wife Jane, who learned to use the dreaded word processor so the manuscript would be done on time; to Natalie Anderson at Brady for her faith and encouragement; and to the folks for whom this book is written—the health care providers who daily strive to provide better care to their patients.

Preface

As a military medic, I learned early on the concept of "CYA," or, loosely translated, "cover your tail." This didn't, by any means, imply that we should cover up mistakes, but rather that all our actions should be well documented. The idea was not just to protect ourselves in the event a case was reviewed, but to provide a good report of our actions so that another medic or physician seeing the patient at a later date would know everything necessary to effectively evaluate any changes in the patient's condition and properly treat the patient. This carried over into civilian life, when as a paramedic I again found myself documenting patient care. When it was my day to drive, I was sometimes asked by other paramedics to trade responsibilities and do the report while they cleaned the blood and vomit off the equipment following a multi-trauma or cardiac arrest call. The reason?

They didn't feel secure that they could get all the necessary, vital information in the small space allocated for it on the run sheet. They recognized that their skills at organizing their ideas and their knowledge of proper terminology and abbreviations were inadequate. I respect those individuals. The scary ones were those whose skills were limited but they didn't recognize it. Those were the ones whose reports you read in dismay, trying to figure out what they found, what the patient had wrong, and what, if anything, they did to treat it. Now, as a Physician's Assistant, I am again placed in the position of being responsible for patient care and documenting every aspect of that care. I again recognize in my peers the desire to do better and to write in a more professional manner. It is to that end that I decided to assemble this pocket reference. It is made to be used by anyone writing a patient care report. It is an assemblage of common tables and charts. It is a list of common abbreviations and their correct, standard meaning. It is a word finder that will enable the user to express him or herself in a manner appropriate to his or her position as a professional health care provider. It is sized so that it will fit in most uniform pockets. Take it with you. It is the partner that knows the correct words to express the condition and care of your patient. It is the friend that will help keep your reports irrefutable in a court of law. Rely on it frequently, that is what it is for.

Todd M. Stanford

Important Numbers

TO CONTACT:

**FREQUENCY/
NUMBER:**

_____ _____

_____ _____

_____ _____

_____ _____

_____ _____

_____ _____

x

TO CONTACT:

FREQUENCY/ NUMBER:

_____   _____

_____   _____

_____   _____

_____   _____

_____   _____

_____   _____

_____   _____

_____   _____

_____   _____

Report
Format

Whether on a surgical ward, in an emergency department, or in the back of an ambulance, if you're involved with patient care, you are probably familiar with writing reports describing patient condition and care. No matter where your contact with the patient occurs, if you write a report describing that contact, you are probably (or should be) using a format of one kind or another. Almost all practitioners of medicine, both military and civilian have adopted use of the "SOAP" format and have used it for decades. In that sense, it has essentially become the standard for documentation. Unfortunately, the "almost all" does not include prehospital care providers. The reason for this is that "SOAP" is a mnemonic representing Subjective, Objective, Assessment and Plan. The

1

assessment portion of this format is where the problem lies. Though EMTs and paramedics are trained to do an accurate, rapid assessment of the patient's condition, they are discouraged repeatedly from "making a diagnosis." They are told to describe a finding, i.e.—"Dextrostix shows less than 25 mg/dl," rather than saying, "The patient appears to be in insulin shock." For this reason, the prehospital care provider often does not report an assessment of the patient's problem, only what he found and what he will do (or did) to care for the patient en route to the medical facility. In order to correct this omission, and to finally bring prehospital care providers under the same standards of documentation of other health care providers, I suggest using the "SOAP" format modified appropriately.

THE MODIFIED SOAP FORMAT

S – Subjective. What the patient or bystanders tell you. This should include anything affecting the reliability of the source. For example, "Bystander stated that patient fell off a bar stool and convulsed for 30 minutes before 911 was called. The bystander had slurred speech and a very strong odor of ETOH." This is where the patient's Chief Complaint and symptoms should be recorded. As you take your history, the information you elicit concerning the patient's problem, whether from him or bystanders, is considered subjective information. Family history that may be related to the patient's problem should also be recorded here: i.e.—"Black male with history of dizzy spells and throbbing headaches complains of epistaxis × 3 hours, uncontrolled with ice and holding nares closed. Patient has family history of stroke and hypertension." Anything the patient attempted to alleviate his problem should be noted as well as the outcome.

A good, short format to follow both while taking and while recording the history is "PQRST": Provocative/Palliative (what makes the problem better or worse); Quality (is the pain or discomfort stabbing, burning, dull, sharp, etc?); Radiating (does the pain go anywhere, shoulder, jaw, down the leg, etc?); Severity ("on a scale of 1 to 10, with 10 being the worst pain you've ever experienced, how does this pain rate?") Also include the source of the patient's "worst pain ever." Time (onset and duration of problem). Any periodicity or sequence with other activity, i.e. eating, sleeping, running, etc. Basically anything you learn from the patient or a bystander (family member, witness, etc.) concerning medical problems, family or social history that is in any way relevant to the present problem needs to go in this section. Tobacco and alcohol use should be recorded here. Additionally, any medical problems or allergies the patient has, and any medications the patient takes regularly is documented here.

O — Objective. This is the section where you record your observations. Dextrostix values, vital signs (not recorded elsewhere on the form), location of obvious deformities, discoloration, edema, unusual angulation of limbs, etc. The cardiac rhythm or dysrhythmia observed on the monitor should be entered here. Evaluations of patient's muscle strength, state of hygiene, mentation, extent and descriptions of obvious damage or injury go here. Unusual odors, actions, or observations of any kind should be well documented. In short, the findings of the physical examination you perform are recorded here. At the scene of an accident, the information concerning mechanism of injury should be presented in this section, as long as you (or your trustworthy partner) made the evaluation. This includes information such as damage to vehicles, distance thrown or fallen, etc.

A — Assessment. This is the often omitted section of the prehospital care report. It is here where the EMT/paramedic documents his impression of the patient's condition. It is here where he says,

"Patient appeared to be in insulin shock. Obvious open fracture of humerus." The key words in the examples are "obvious" and "appeared." No one expects you to have the diagnostic expertise of a physician; but if the patient has a dextrostix of less than 25 mg/dl and snoring respirations, and after you have administered an amp of D50 he regains conciousness and asks why you're in his bedroom, it's pretty safe to say his problem was insulin shock. If you truly have no idea what the patient's problem is, at least summarize your impression of the patient's problem: i.e. — "Patient appears to be in severe epigastric pain." Get in the habit of putting SOMETHING (as long as it is accurate) in this section.

P — Plan. This is where you should describe in explicit detail every aspect of the patient's management. For example: "Two large bore IVs of Ringer's Lactate were established in the bilateral antecubital fossae and run wide open. Patient was immobilized with a nec loc, a KED was applied, and the patient was removed from the car and strapped to a backboard. CID was added for additional immobilization of the C-spine and oxygen was administered via non-rebreathing face mask at a rate of 16 Lpm." Document everything you did to manage the patient. The one thing you leave out may be the thing that returns to haunt you months or even years later. Even though you properly managed your patient, if you did not document a specific procedure or action, it is assumed you didn't do it. What's worse, you can't prove you did!

Chronology: Whether recording the patient's history or your care of the patient, maintain chronological order. Make your report easy to read by following a logical sequence when listing events. Don't say you immobilized the C-spine with a CID before you document placing the patient on a backboard. Get in the habit of recalling in your mind, then recording on paper, each event that occurred, as it occurred, from the time you arrived on the scene. In the subjective portion, say that the patient fell on ice two weeks ago and felt a sharp pain in his arm which has gotten progressively worse. Now, he can't move his fingers. Don't say, "The patient noticed that he couldn't move his fingers when he got out of bed today," then as an afterthought, "Patient fell two weeks ago." Keep it simple but thorough and keep it in the order that the events actually occurred.

Problem Orientation: You are not writing an admission history and physical as would be done by

6

a resident. You are concisely describing your inter-
actions with the patient. Keep focused on the information related to the patient's present problem. The fact that the patient smokes three packs
of cigarettes a day is irrelevant if he is being trans-
ported for a lacerated foot. On the other hand; if
that same patient called because he began "coughing differently than usual two weeks ago," and
now he is coughing up blood, that is an extremely
important part of his social history that needs to
be both reported to the ED en route and documented in your report. Reports are notoriously
short of space when the patient is seriously ill or
injured. Like your physical examination, your report should focus on the patient's present problem. It should be problem oriented.

Pertinency: Just as your report should be problem oriented, it should contain all the pertinents.
Both positive and negative responses and findings
that are pertinent to the patient's present problem
should be listed. For our friend with the cut foot
it isn't really necessary to report your findings on
auscultation of his lungs. That isn't pertinent to
his present problem. Once he starts coughing up
blood, however, the fact that there are fine rales
in the base of his left lung is just as important (pertinent) as the fact that he has coarse rales, rhonchi

and expiratory wheezes in all fields of his right lung. These findings indicate that he has a major problem with his right lung that has not yet involved his left one as extensively, if at all. Therefore these are both pertinent positives and negatives that must be documented. In short, whether a finding is normal or abnormal, positive or negative, if it is pertinent to the patient's problem, document it.

Redundancy: As was noted earlier, space is often short on the typical "run sheet." For this reason, unless local procedures dictate otherwise, if you list an objective finding elsewhere on the form, don't repeat it in the body of the SOAP format. It usually isn't necessary. Exceptions to this are when you list drugs or fluids administered in a separate block on the form. You still need to document the order, times, routes and amounts of medication administered. Changes in cardiac rhythms, vitals, levels of consciousness, etc., though listed elsewhere, should be repeated in the body of the report. Other than those situations which need to more clearly show a cause and effect relationship chronologically, repetition of information found elsewhere in the report is redundant and unnecessary.

Common Abbreviations

ā	Before
abd.	Abdomen
abs.	Absent
AD	Right ear
add.	Adduction
ADL	Activities of daily living
admin.	Administer(ed)
A fib.	Atrial fibrillation
AgNO₃	Silver Nitrate
A.M.	Morning
AMA	Against Medical Advice
AMI	Acute myocardial infarction
amp	Ampule
Amp.	Amputation

amt.	Amount
ant	Anterior
appt.	Appointment
AS	Left ear
ASA	Aspirin
ASAP	As soon as possible
AU	Both ears
AV Node	Atrioventricular node
BaE	Barium enema
BC	Birth control
BCP	Birth control pills
b.i.d.	Twice a day
bilat	Bilateral
BM	Bowel movement
BP	Blood pressure
br. snds.	Breath sounds
BS	Bowel sounds
C	Cervical
cc.	Cubic centimeter
$\bar{c}$	With
CA	Cancer
Ca	Calcium
CABG ("cabbage")	Coronary artery bypass graft

CAD	Coronary artery disease
cal.	Caliber
CBC	Complete blood count
CC	Chief complaint
CHF	Congestive heart failure
cl.	Clear
cm.	Centimeter
cm^3	Cubic centimeter
CNS	Central nervous system
CO_2	Carbon dioxide
CO	Carbon monoxide
COLD	Chronic obstructed lung disease
c/o	Complains of
conc.	Concentration
cond.	Condition
COPD	Chronic obstructive pulmonary disease
CPR	Cardiopulmonary resuscitation
crit, crt.	Hematocrit
CSF	Cerebral spinal fluid
CVA	Cerebrovascular accident
CXR	Chest X-ray

d	Day
DBP	Diastolic blood pressure
D/C	Discontinue
D&C	Dilation and curettage
Deform.	Deformity
degen.	Degenerative
Derm.	Dermatology
DI	Diabetes insipidus
dig.	Digitalis
disloc.	Dislocated
DM	Diabetes Mellitus
DMSO	Dimethyl sulfoxide
DOB	Date of birth
DOE	Dyspnea on exertion
dsg.	Dressing
DTR	Deep tendon reflexes
DT's	Delerium tremens
Dx	Diagnosis
ea.	Each
EBL	Estimated blood loss
ECG	Electrocardiogram
ED	Emergency department
EDC	Estimated date of confinement

EDD	Estimated date of delivery
EEG	Electroencephalogram
e.g.	For example
EKG	Electrocardiogram
ENT	Ear, nose & throat
EP	Ectopic pregnancy
Epi.	Epinephrine
ETA	Estimated time of arrival
ET	Endotracheal
ETH	Elixir terpin hydrate
etiol.	Etiology
ETOH	Drinking alcohol
exam	Examination
F	Fahrenheit
FB	Foreign body
Fe	Iron
fem.	Femoral
FH	Family History
fl.	Fluid
flex.	Flexion
freq.	Frequency, frequent
FROM	Full range of motion
ft.	Foot, feet
FTND	Full term normal delivery

FTT	Failure to thrive
f/u	Follow up
FUO	Fever of unknown origin
FWB	Full weight bearing
Fx	Fracture
g	Gram
ga.	Gauge
gal.	Gallon
GB	Gallbladder
GC	Gonorrhea
gd.	Good
gen.	General
Ger.	Geriatric
GF	Grandfather
GG	Gamma globulin
GI	Gastrointestinal
gl.	Gland
gluc.	Glucose
GM	Grandmother
GM seizure	Grand mal seizure
GNID	Gram negative intercellular diplococci
gr.	Grain
grav.	Gravida

GSW	Gunshot wound
GTT	Glucose tolerance test
gtts.	Drops
GU	Genitourinary
Gyn.	Gynecology
h	Hour
HA	Headache
Hb.	Hemoglobin
HBO	Hyperbaric oxygen
HC	Hydrocortisone
HCG	Human chorionic gonadotropin
Hct.	Hematocrit
HCTZ	Hydrochlorothiazide
HDL	High density lipoproteins
Hg	Mercury
Hgb.	Hemoglobin
HIV	Human immunodeficiency virus
HNP	Herniated nucleus pulposus
h/o	History of
H_2O	Water
H_2O_2	Hydrogen peroxide
H & P	History and physical

HPI	History of present illness
HR	Heart rate
HS	Heart sounds
h.s.	At bedtime
HTN	Hypertension
husb.	Husband
Hx	History
I	Iodine
IC	Intracranial, intracardiac
ICM	Intercostal margin
ICP	Intracranial pressure
ICS	Intercostal space
ID	Identify (identification)
I & D	Incision and drainage
IM	Intramuscular
inf.	Infant, infection
info.	Information
inj.	Injury
ins.	Insurance
int.	Internal
I&O	Intake and output
IPPB	Intermittent positive pressure breathing
IR	Infra red

irreg.	Irregular
IU	International unit
IUD	Intrauterine device
IV	Intravenous
IVPB	Intravenous piggyback
J.	Joule
jaund.	Jaundice
jct.	Junction
JR	Junctional rhythm
JVD	Jugular venous distention
K	Potassium
KA	Ketoacidosis
KCl	Potassium chloride
kg.	Kilogram
km.	Kilometer
KOH	Potassium hydroxide
KVO	Keep vein open
L.	Liter
Ⓛ	Left
lac.	Laceration
LASER	Light amplification by the stimulated emission of radiation
lat.	Lateral

LB	Lower back
lb.	Pound
LBBB	Left bundle branch block
LBP	Low back pain
L & D	Labor and delivery
LD_{50}	Lethal dose to 50% of test population
LDL	Low density lipoproteins
lg.	Large
LHF	Left heart failure
Li	Lithium
lig.	Ligament
liq.	Liquid
LLQ	Left lower quadrant
LMP	Last menstrual period
LNMP	Last normal menstrual period
LOC	Loss (or level) of conciousness
LOM	Loss (or limit) of motion
LP	Lumbar puncture
LPN	Licensed practical nurse
LS	Lumbosacral
LSB	Left sternal border
LUQ	Left upper quadrant

m.	Meter
mand.	Mandible
MAST	Military (or medical) anti-shock trousers
McB. pt.	McBurney's point
mcg.	Microgram
MCL	Midclavicular line
med.	Medial
mEq.	Milliequivalent
mets.	Metastases
M & F	Mother and father
Mg	Magnesium
mg.	Milligram
$MgSO_4$	Magnesium sulfate
MI	Myocardial infarction
misc.	Miscellaneous
ML	Midline
ml.	Milliliter
mm.	Millimeter
mm^3	Cubic millimeter
mo.	Month
mod.	Moderate
MOM	Milk of magnesia
Mono.	Infectious mononucleosis

mos.	Months
MS	Morphine sulfate
MSL	Midsternal line
multip.	Multiparous
musc.	Muscle
N.	Nerve
NA	Not applicable (available)
Na	Sodium
NaCl	Sodium Chloride
NAD	No acute distress
$NaHCO_3$	Sodium bicarbonate
narc.	Narcotic
nas.	Nasal
nat.	Natural
neg.	Negative
Neuro.	Neurology
NG	Nasogastric
NM	Neuromuscular
NMI	No middle initial
norm.	Normal
NP	Nasopharyngeal
NPI	No present illness
NPO	Nothing by mouth
NS	Normal saline

NSAID	Nonsteroidal anti-inflammatory drug
NSR	Normal sinus rhythm
NSU	Nonspecific urethritis
NT	Nasotracheal
NTG	Nitroglycerin
NTP	Nitroprusside
N & V	Nausea and vomiting
NVD	Nausea, vomiting, diarrhea
NV	Neurovascular
NWB	Nonweight bearing
O_2	Oxygen
ō	None, no
OB	Obstetrics
Ob/Gyn	Obstetrics/gynecology
obl.	Oblique
occ.	Occasional
OD	Right eye
OD.	Overdose
oper.	Operation
Ophth.	Ophthalmology
OR	Operating room
ORIF	Open reduction, internal fixation

orig.	Original
Ortho.	Orthopedics
OS	Left eye
OTC	Over the counter
OU	Both eyes
oz.	Ounce
$\bar{p}$	After
PA	Physician's Assistant
PAL	Posterior axillary line
palp.	Palpable
palpit.	Palpitations
parox.	Paroxysmal
pass.	Passive
PAT	Paroxysmal atrial tachycardia
Pb	Lead
PCN	Penicillin
p/d	Packs (cigarettes) per day
PDR	Physician's desk reference
PE	Physical examination, pulmonary embolus
PEARL	Pupils equal and reactive to light
Peds.	Pediatrics

PEEP	Positive end expiratory pressure
per	By order of
per.	Period
perf.	Perforated
perm.	Permanent
pers.	Personal
PID	Pelvic inflammatory disease
PJC	Premature junctional contraction
PKU	Phenylketonuria
P.M.	Afternoon
PMH	Past medical history
PMS	Premenstrual syndrome
PND	Paroxysmal nocturnal dyspnea
pneumo	Pneumothorax
p.o.	By mouth
POD	Post operative day
PODx	Post operative diagnosis
poplit.	Popliteal
Pos.	Position
poss.	Possible

post.	Posterior
ppm	Parts per million
PR	Pulse rate
pr.	Pair
p.r.	Administer rectally
preg.	Pregnant
prelim.	Preliminary
premie	Premature infant
prenat.	Prenatal
preop.	Preoperative
prep.	Prepare
press.	Pressure
prev.	Previous
PRN	As necessary
PROM	Premature rupture of membranes
pron.	Pronation
prox.	Proximal
psi	Pounds per square inch
PSVT	Paroxysmal supraventricular tachycardia
pt.	Patient
PUD	Peptic ulcer disease
pulm.	Pulmonary

PVC	Premature ventricular contraction
PVD	Peripheral vascular disease
PWB	Partial weight bearing
q.	Each
q.a.m.	Each morning
q.d.	Each day
q.h.	Each hour
q.4h.	Every four hours
q.i.d.	Four times a day
qt.	Quart
R	Rate
®	Right
RBBB	Right bundle branch block
reconstr.	Reconstruction
rect.	Rectal
ref.	Reference
reg.	Region
rehab.	Rehabilitation
rel.	Relative
rem.	Remove
resp.	Respirations
ret.	Retired
RHD	Rheumatic heart disease

RHF	Right heart failure
RL	Ringer's lactate
RLL	Right lower lobe
RLQ	Right lower quadrant
RML	Right middle lobe
RMSF	Rocky mountain spotted fever
RN	Registered nurse
R/O	Rule out
ROM	Range of motion
ROS	Review of systems
rot.	Rotate (rotating)
RSB	Right sternal border
RUL	Right upper lobe
RUQ	Right upper quadrant
Rx	Medication
S	Son
$\bar{s}$	Without
sal.	Saline
SBE	Subacute bacterial endocarditis
SBP	Systolic blood pressure
SC	Sickle cell
SD	Sudden death

sect.	Section
sev.	Several
SIDS	Sudden infant death syndrome
SIW	Self-inflicted wound
SL	Sublingual
sl.	Slight
SLE	Systemic lupus erythematosus
sm.	Small
SNS	Sympathetic nervous system
SOB	Short of breath
soln.	Solution
SOP	Standard operating procedure
SP	Systolic pressure
sp.cd.	Spinal cord
spont.	Spontaneous
SQ	Subcutaneous
S & S	Signs and symptoms
ST	Sinus tachycardia
STAT	Immediately
STD	Sexually transmitted disease
std.	Standard
stim.	Stimulus
sup.	Superior

supp.	Suppository
Surg.	Surgery or surgeon
susp.	Suspension
SVT	Supraventricular tachycardia
sym.	Symmetrical
T	Temperature
tab.	Tablet
TB	Tuberculosis
TC	Throat culture
TCA	Terminal cancer
TCN	Tetracycline
TIA	Transient ischemic attack
t.i.d.	Three times a day
tinct.	Tincture
TKO	To keep open
TLC	Tender loving care
TM	Tympanic membrane
TMJ	Temporomandibular joint
T/O	Telephone order
tol.	Tolerate(d)
top.	Topical
TP	Syphilis
trach.	Tracheostomy
tract.	Traction

trans.	Transverse
Tx	Treatment
UGI	Upper gastrointestinal series
UHF	Ultra high frequency
unilat.	Unilateral
URI	Upper respiratory infection
UT	Urinary tract
UTI	Urinary tract infection
UV	Ultraviolet
V.	Vein
VA	Veteran's administration
vac.	Vacuum
vasc.	Vascular
VD	Venereal disease
V fib.	Ventricular fibrillation
vert.	Vertical
V/O	Verbal order
vol.	Volume
VR	Ventricular rate
vs.	Versus
vss.	Vital signs
VT	Ventricular tachycardia
WBC	White blood count
wk.	Week

WNL	Within normal limits.
	We never looked.
WPW	Wolf-Parkinson-White
wr.	Wrist
wt.	Weight
X	Times
X-fer	Transfer
yel.	Yellow
y.o.	Years old
yr.	Year
$\simeq$	Approximately
@	At
Δ	Change
$\downarrow$	Decrease
$=$	Equal
$\female$	Female
$>$	Greater than
$\uparrow$	Increase
$<$	Less than
$\male$	Male
$\ominus$	Negative, absent
/	Per
$\oplus$	Positive, present

Common Abbreviations

Absent	abs.
Abdomen	abd.
Activities of daily living	ADL
Acute myocardial infarction	AMI
Adduction	add.
Administer(ed)	admin.
Administer rectally	p.r.
After	$\bar{p}$
Afternoon	P.M.
Against medical advice	AMA
Amount	amt.
Ampule	amp
Amputation	amp.

Anterior	ant
Appointment	appt.
Approximately	≃
As necessary	PRN
As soon as possible	ASAP
Aspirin	ASA
At	@
At bedtime	h.s.
Atrial fibrillation	A fib.
Atrioventricular node	AV Node
Barium enema	BaE
Before	$\bar{a}$
Bilateral	bilat
Birth control	BC
Birth control pills	BCP
Blood pressure	BP
Both ears	AU
Both eyes	OU
Bowel movement	BM
Bowel sounds	BS
Breath sounds	br. snds.
By mouth	p.o.
By order of	per
Calcium	Ca

Caliber	cal.
Cancer	CA
Carbon dioxide	CO_2
Carbon monoxide	CO
Cardiopulmonary resuscitation	CPR
Centimeter	cm.
Central nervous system	CNS
Cerebral spinal fluid	CSF
Cerebrovascular accident	CVA
Cervical	C
Change	Δ
Chest x-ray	CXR
Chief complaint	CC
Chronic obstructed lung disease	COLD
Chronic obstructive pulmonary disease	COPD
Clear	cl.
Complains of	c/o
Complete blood count	CBC
Concentration	conc.
Condition	cond.
Congestive heart failure	CHF

Coronary artery bypass graft	CABG ("cabbage")
Coronary artery disease	CAD
Cubic centimeter	cc.
Cubic centimeter	cm³
Date of birth	DOB
Day	d
Decrease	↓
Deep tendon reflexes	DTR
Deformity	Deform.
Degenerative	degen.
Delirium tremens	DTs
Dermatology	Derm.
Diabetes Insipidous	DI
Diabetes Mellitus	DM
Diagnosis	Dx
Diastolic blood pressure	DBP
Digitalis	dig.
Dilation and curettage	D & C
Dimethyl sulfoxide	DMSO
Discontinue	D/C
Dislocated	disloc.
Dressing	dsg.
Drinking alcohol	ETOH

Drops	gtts.
Dyspnea on exertion	DOE
Each	ea.
Each	q
Each day	q.d.
Each hour	q.h.
Each morning	q.A.M.
Ear, nose & throat	ENT
Ectopic pregnancy	EP
Electrocardiogram	ECG
Electrocardiogram	EKG
Electroencephalogram	EEG
Elixir terpin hydrate	ETH
Emergency department	ED
Endotracheal	ET
Epinephrine	epi.
Equal	=
Estimated blood loss	EBL
Estimated date of confine-ment	EDC
Estimated date of delivery	EDD
Estimated time of arrival	ETA
Etiology	etiol.
Every four hours	q.4h.

Examination	exam
Fahrenheit	F.
Failure to thrive	FTT
Family history	FH
Female	♀
Femoral	fem.
Fever of unknown origin	FUO
Flexion	flex.
Fluid	fl.
Follow up	f/u
Foot, feet	ft.
For example	e.g.
Foreign body	FB
Four times a day	q.i.d.
Fracture	Fx
Frequency, frequent	freq
Full range of motion	FROM
Full term normal delivery	FTND
Full weight bearing	FWB
Gallbladder	GB
Gallon	gal.
Gamma globulin	GG
Gastrointestinal	GI
Gauge	ga.

General	gen.
Genitourinary	GU
Geriatric	Ger.
Gland	gl.
Glucose	gluc.
Grain	gr.
Gonorrhea	GC
Good	gd
Gram	g
Gram negative intercellular diplococci	GNID
Grandfather	GF
Grand Mal seizure	GM seizure
Grandmother	GM
Gravida	grav.
Greater than	>
Gunshot wound	GSW
Gynecology	Gyn.
Headache	HA
Heart rate	HR
Heart sound	HS
Hematocrit	Hct.
Hematocrit	crit, crt.
Hemoglobin	Hb.

Hemoglobin	Hgb.
Herniated nucleus pulposus	HNP
High density lipoproteins	HDL
History	Hx
History and physical	H & P
History of	h/o
History of present illness	HPI
Hour	h
Human chorionic gonado-tropin	HCG
Human immunodeficiency virus	HIV
Husband	husb.
Hydrochlorothiazide	HCTZ
Hydrocortisone	HC
Hydrogen peroxide	H_2O_2
Hyperbaric oxygen	HBO
Hypertension	HTN
Identify (identification)	ID
Immediately	STAT
Incision and drainage	I & D
Increase	↑
Infant, infection	inf.
Infectious mononucleosis	Mono

Infra red	IR
Information	info.
Injury	inj.
Insurance	ins.
Intake and output	I & O
Intercostal margin	ICM
Intercostal space	ICS
Intermittent positive pressure breathing	IPPB
Internal	int
International unit	IU
Intracranial, intracardiac	IC
Intracranial pressure	ICP
Intramuscular	IM
Intrauterine device	IUD
Intravenous	IV
Intravenous piggyback	IVPB
Iodine	I
Iron	Fe
Irregular	irreg.
Jaundice	Jaund.
Joule	J.
Jugular venous distention	JVD
Junction	Jct.

Junctional rhythm	JR
Keep vein open	KVO
Ketoacidosis	KA
Kilogram	Kg.
Kilometer	km.
Labor and delivery	L & D
Laceration	lac.
Large	lg.
Last menstrual period	LMP
Last normal menstrual period	LNMP
Lateral	lat
Lead	Pb
Left	Ⓛ
Left bundle branch block	LBBB
Left ear	AS
Left eye	OS
Left heart failure	LHF
Left lower quadrant	LLQ
Left sternal border	LSB
Left upper quadrant	LUQ
Less than	<
Lethal dose to 50% of test population	LD_{50}
Licensed practical nurse	LPN

Ligament	lig.
Light amplification by the stimulated emission of radiation	LASER
Liquid	liq.
Liter	L.
Lithium	Li.
Loss (or level) of consciousness	LOC
Loss (or limit) of motion	LOM
Low back pain	LBP
Low density lipoproteins	LDL
Lower back	LB
Lumbar puncture	LP
Lumbosacral	LS
Magnesium	Mg
Magnesium sulfate	$MgSO_4$
Male	♂
Mandible	Mand.
Military (or medical) anti-shock trousers	MAST
McBurney's point	McB. pt.
Medial	med
Medication	Rx

Mercury	Hg
Metastases	mets.
Meter	m.
Microgram	mcg
Midclavicular line	MCL
Midline	ML
Midsternal line	MSL
Milk of magnesia	MOM
Milliequivalent	mEq
Milligram	mg
Milliliter	ml.
Millimeter	mm
Miscellaneous	misc.
Moderate	mod
Month	mo.
Months	mos.
Morning	A.M.
Morphine sulfate	MS
Mother and father	M & F
Multiparous	multip
Muscle	musc.
Myocardial infarction	MI
Narcotic	narc.
Nasal	nas.

Nasogastric	NG
Nasopharyngeal	NP
Nasotracheal	NT
Natural	nat
Nausea and vomiting	N & V
Nausea, vomiting, diarrhea	NVD
Negative	neg
Negative, absent	$\ominus$
Nerve	N.
Neurology	Neuro.
Neuromuscular	NM
Neurovascular	NV
Nitroglycerin	NTG
Nitroprusside	NTP
No acute distress	NAD
No middle initial	NMI
No present illness	NPI
None, No	$\bar{o}$
Nonspecific urethritis	NSU
Nonsteroidal anti-inflammatory drug	NSAID
Nonweight bearing	NWB
Normal	norm.
Normal saline	NS

Normal sinus rhythm	NSR
Not applicable (available)	NA
Nothing by mouth	NPO
Oblique	obl.
Obstetrics	OB
Obstetrics/gynecology	Ob/Gyn
Occasional	occ.
Open reduction, internal fixation	ORIF
Operating room	OR
Operation	oper.
Ophthalmology	Ophth.
Original	orig
Orthopedics	Ortho.
Ounce	oz.
Overdose	OD
Over the counter	OTC
Oxygen	O_2
Packs (cigarettes) per day	p/d
Pair	pr
Palpable	palp
Palpitations	palpit
Paroxysmal	parox
Paroxysmal atrial tachycardia	PAT

Paroxysmal nocturnal dyspnea	PND
Paroxysmal supraventricular tachycardia	PSVT
Parts per million	ppm
Partial weight bearing	PWB
Passive	pass.
Past medical history	PMH
Patient	pt.
Pediatrics	peds.
Pelvic inflammatory disease	PID
Penicillin	PCN
Peptic ulcer disease	PUD
Per	/
Perforated	perf.
Period	per.
Peripheral vascular disease	PVD
Permanent	perm.
Personal	pers
Phenylketonuria	PKU
Physical examination/ pulmonary embolus	PE
Physician's Assistant	PA
Physician's Desk Reference	PDR

Pneumothorax	pneumo
Popliteal	poplit.
Position	Pos
Positive, present	⊕
Positive end expiratory pressure	PEEP
Possible	poss
Posterior	post
Posterior axillary line	PAL
Post operative day	POD
Post operative diagnosis	PODx
Potassium	K
Potassium chloride	KCl
Potassium hydroxide	KOH
Pound	lb.
Pounds per square inch	psi
Pregnant	preg
Preliminary	prelim
Premature infant	premie
Premature junctional contraction	PJC
Premature rupture of membranes	PROM

Premature ventricular contraction	PVC
Premenstrual syndrome	PMS
Prenatal	prenat
Preoperative	preop.
Prepare	prep
Pressure	press
Previous	prev.
Pronation	pron.
Proximal	prox.
Pulmonary	pulm.
Pulse rate	PR
Pupils equal and reactive to light	PEARL
Quart	qt.
Range of motion	ROM
Rate	R
Reconstruction	reconst.
Rectal	rect.
Reference	ref.
Region	reg.
Registered nurse	RN
Rehabilitation	rehab.

Relative	rel.
Remove	rem.
Respirations	resp.
Retired	ret.
Review of systems	ROS
Rheumatic heart disease	RHD
Right	®
Right bundle branch block	RBBB
Right ear	AD
Right eye	OD
Right heart failure	RHF
Right lower lobe	RLL
Right lower quadrant	RLQ
Right middle lobe	RML
Right sternal border	RSB
Ringer's lactate	RL
Rocky Mountain spotted fever	RMSF
Rotate (rotating)	rot.
Rule out	R/O
Saline	NaCl
Section	sect.
Self-inflicted wound	SIW

Several	sev.
Sexually transmitted disease	STD
Short of breath	SOB
Sickle cell	SC
Signs and symptoms	S & S
Silver Nitrate	AgNO$_3$
Sinus tachycardia	ST
Slight	sl.
Small	sm.
Sodium	Na
Sodium Bicarbonate	NaHCO$_3$
Sodium chloride	NaCl
Solution	soln.
Son	S
Spinal cord	sp.cd.
Spontaneous	spont.
Standard	std.
Standard operating procedure	SOP
Stimulus	stim.
Subacute bacterial endocarditis	SBE
Subcutaneous	SQ
Sublingual	SL

Sudden death	SD
Sudden infant death syndrome	SIDS
Superior	sup.
Suppository	supp.
Supraventricular tachycardia	SVT
Surgery or surgeon	Surg.
Suspension	susp.
Sympathetic nervous system	SNS
Symmetrical	sym.
Syphilis	TP
Systemic lupus erythematosus	SLE
Systolic blood pressure	SBP
Systolic pressure	SP
Tablet	tab.
Telephone order	T/O
Temperature	temp.
Temporomandibular joint	TMJ
Tender loving care	TLC
Terminal cancer	TCA
Tetracycline	TCN
Three times a day	t.i.d.
Times	X
Throat culture	TC

Tincture	tinct.
To keep open	TKO
Tolerate(d)	tol.
Topical	top.
Tracheostomy	trach.
Traction	tract.
Transfer	X-fer
Transient ischemic attack	TIA
Transverse	trans.
Treatment	Tx
Tuberculosis	TB
Twice a day	b.i.d.
Tympanic membrane	TM
Ultra high frequency	UHF
Ultraviolet	UV
Unilateral	unilat.
Upper gastrointestinal series	UGI
Upper respiratory infection	URI
Urinary tract	UT
Urinary tract infection	UTI
Vacuum	vac.
Vascular	vasc.
Vein	V.
Venereal disease	VD

Ventricular fibrillation	V fib.
Ventricular rate	VR
Ventricular tachycardia	VT
Verbal order	V/O
Versus	vs.
Vertical	vert.
Veteran's administration	VA
Vital signs	vss
Volume	vol.
Water	H_2O
Week	wk.
Weight	wt.
White blood count	WBC
With	$\bar{c}$
Within normal limits	WNL
Without	$\bar{s}$
Wolf-Parkinson-White	WPW
Wrist	wr.
Year	yr.
Years old	y.o.
Yellow	yel.

Word
Finder

Abnormally high temperature	Hyperthermic
Abnormally low temperature	Hypothermic
Air hunger	Dyspnea
Air (free) in abdomen	Pneumoperitoneum
Air (free) in thorax	Pneumothorax
Air (free) under skin	Subcutaneous emphysema
Appetite, absent	Anorexia
Appetite, insatiable	Hyperorexia
Belly button	Umbilicus
Bleed to death, remove all blood	Exsanguinate
Blood clot, vascular, moving	Embolus

Blood clot, vascular, stationary	Thrombus
Blood clot, within tissue/body space	Hematoma
Blood in abdomen (abdominal cavity)	Hemoperitoneum
Blood in pericardial sac	Hemopericardium
Blood in stool (bloody)	Hematochezia
Blood in stool (tarry)	Melena
Blood in thorax (pleural cavity)	Hemothorax
Blood in urine	Hematuria
Blood poisoning	Lymphangitis
Blood pressure, high	Hypertension
Blood pressure, low	Hypotension
Bloodshot eyes	Injected conjunctiva
Blood, spitting	Hemoptysis
Blood, vomiting	Hematemesis
Both sides	Bilateral
Break	Fracture
Bruise	Contusion
Burping, belching	Eructation
Chickenpox	Varicella

Cut, jagged edges	Laceration
Cut, smooth edges	Incision
Cut, layers of skin scraped away	Abrasion
Cut, segment of tissue torn away	Avulsion
Discoloration	Ecchymosis
Double vision	Diplopia
Earache	Otalgia
Ear, discharge from	Otorrhea
Ear infection, inner ear	Otitis media
Ear infection, outer ear	Otitis externa
Ear, ringing in	Tinnitis
Earwax	Cerumen
Eating, increased	Polyphagia
Examine, by tapping	Percussion
Examine, by touching	Palpation
Examine, using a stethoscope	Auscultation
Extra in number	Supernumerary
Feverish, temperature >100 degrees F.	Febrile
Fever, lack of, normothermic	Afebrile
Fit, convulsions	Seizure activity

Foul breath	Halitosis
Foul smelling	Fetid
Gallbladder disease	Cholecystitis
Gallstone	Cholelith
Headache	Cephalgia
Heartburn	Pyrosis
Hives	Urticaria
Hunchback	Kyphosis
Indigestion	Dyspepsia
Infected hair follicle	Furuncle
Intercourse, painful	Dyspareunia
Inability to move arms	Superior paraplegia
Inability to move any limb	Quadriplegia
Inability to move limbs — one side	Hemiplegia
Inability to move lower extremities	Paraplegia
Inability to move one leg	Hemiparaplegia
Inability to speak	Aphasic
Itching	Pruritis
Jaundice, Jaundiced	Icterus, Icteric
Kidney stone	Nephrolith

Kneecap	Patella
Measles	Rubeola
Measles, German, three day	Rubella
Menstruation, absent	Amenorrhea
Menstruation, first	Menarche
Menstruation, painful	Dysmenor-rhea
Menstruation, unusually heavy	Menorrhagia
Nasal discharge	Rhinorrhea
Nosebleed	Epistaxis
Opening, hole	Aperture, orifice
Opposite side	Contralateral
Orogenital stimulation	Fellatio
Pain — joint	Arthralgia
Pain — muscle	Myalgia
Passing gas from rectum	Flatulent
Piles	Hemorrhoids
Pounding heartbeat (symptom)	Palpitations
Rash	Cutaneous eruption
Redness, inflamed	Erythematous
Same side	Ipsilateral

Scratches, from scratching an itch	Excoriations
Sensation, absence of	Anesthesia
Sensation, tingling, burning	Paresthesia
Sex drive	Libido
Shingles	Herpes Zoster
Shoulder blade	Scapula
Sneezing	Tarmus
Snoring	Stertorous
Stomach growls	Borborygmus
Swallowing, difficulty	Dysphagia
Swelling — joints	Effusion
Swelling — soft tissue	Edema
Thirst, excessive	Polydipsia
Throbbing	Pulsatile
Toothache	Odontalgia
Urination, excessive	Polyuria
Urination, painful, burning, difficult	Dysuria
Urine, pus present	Pyuria
Vomit	Emesis
Watering eyes, excessive tearing	Epiphoria
Whooping cough	Pertussis

EMS
Terminology

A

A-Pillar   The first pillar (at the windshield) of a vehicle, between the roof and vehicle body.

Abandonment   Termination of care without either the consent of the patient, or without transferring care to an equally or more qualified EMS provider.

Abdomen   The body cavity whose boundaries are the diaphragm and the rim of the pelvis.

Abduct   Movement away from the midline.

Abrasion   Wound caused by scraping or scratching away the skin.

Abscess   A collection of pus surrounded by inflamed tissue.

Accommodation Changing the shape of the eye's lens to focus on an object.

Acidosis Abnormally low (<7.35) blood pH.

Acute Having rapid onset and short duration.

Adduct Movement towards the midline.

Afebrile Without fever.

Affect Manifestation of mood.

Agonal Pertaining to dying.

Akinetic Inability to move.

Alkalosis Abnormally high (>7.45) blood pH.

Alzheimer's Disease A degenerative disorder whose latter stage is characterized by increasing dementia.

Amenorrhea Abnormal absence of menses.

Amnesia Loss of memory.

Amniotic Sac "Bag of water," the membrane that contains the fetus surrounded by amniotic fluid.

Amputation Removal of an appendage. Can be complete or partial, surgical or traumatic, depending on circumstances.

Analgesic Medication taken for the relief of pain.

Anaphylactic Reaction Severe allergic reaction that can lead to profound shock and death if untreated.

Anastomosis Surgical union of hollow structures such as blood vessels. Also refers to reconnection of nerves.

Anemia Inadequate concentration of oxygen transporting material in a given volume of blood.

Anesthesia Loss of sensation.

Aneurysm Abnormally dilated portion of an artery.

Angle of Louis Junction of the manubrium and body of the sternum.

Anorexia Loss of appetite.

Anterior Front or ventral portion of the body.

Anuretic Inability to urinate.

Aphonic Inability to speak.

Apnea Absence of breathing.

Apneic Not breathing.

Arthralgia Joint pain.

Arthritis Inflammation of a joint.

Articulation Point where two bones touch the joint.

Artifact Manifestation of electronic "noise," or interference, on an EKG tracing.

Ascites Abnormal accumulation of fluid in the abdomen.

Aseptic Sterile.

Asphyxiation Death caused by lack of oxygen. Suffocation.

Aspirate Inhalation of non-gaseous material into the lung. Also to apply a vacuum.

Asthma Narrowing of the airways in response to an irritant or allergen.

Asthenia Weakness or disability.

Ataxia Absence or loss of coordination.

Atrophy Wasting away of body tissues or the entire body.

Aura Sensory hallucination preceding seizure activity.

Auricle External ear.

Auscultation Examine by listening with a stethoscope.

Autonomic Nervous System The system which controls body processes without requiring conscious thought or effort.

Avulsion Partial or complete removal of a flap of skin.

Axilla The armpit.

B

B-Pillar The second support pillar from the windshield between the vehicle's body and roof.

Bale Hook Short metal hook with a handle arranged perpendicular to the shank. Originally used to manipulate bales of hay or rags, it now has various rescue applications.

Bandage Material used to hold a dressing in place.

Barotrauma Injury caused by changes in ambient pressure such as incurred while diving or flying.

Battle's Sign Ecchymosis over the mastoid process (behind the ear). One indication of a basilar skull fracture.

Bends Diver's jargon for decompression sickness. Caused by nitrogen bubbles in body tissue.

Bifurcation Dividing or forking into two branches.

Bilateral Referring to both sides.

Biologic Death Brain death. Traditionally thought to occur about six to ten minutes after clinical death.

Biparous Delivery Delivery of twins.

Blanch Lose color; become pale.

Bloody Show Vaginal discharge of blood tinged mucous that signals the onset of labor.

Bolus A single mass of a substance (usually relatively large) for injection or ingestion.

Borborygmus Rumbling bowel sounds that can be heard at a distance from the patient. "Stomach growling."

Bounding Unusually strong. Usually used in reference to a pulse.

Bradycardia Abnormally slow heart rate (<60 beats/minute).

Bradypnea Abnormally slow respiration (<12 breaths/minute).

Breech Birth/Presentation Vaginal delivery during which the presenting part of the fetus is some body part other than the head.

Bruit Abnormal harsh or musical intermittent sound auscultated over a blood vessel, caused by turbulent flow of blood.

Buccal Pertaining to the cheek, particularly the oral mucosa.

C

C-Pillar The third pillar between the roof and body of a vehicle counting from the front. The pillar at the windshield is number 1—the A pillar.

Carbon Dioxide (CO_2) colorless, odorless gas that is a byproduct of aerobic metabolism.

Carbon Monoxide (CO) colorless odorless, toxic gas produced by the inefficient oxidation of carbon compounds.

Cardiac Pertaining to the heart.

Cardiomegaly Enlarged heart.

Caries Necrosis of teeth; cavities.

Carina Bifurcation of the trachea into the left and right main stem bronchi.

Carbuncle Skin infection characterized by interconnected, subcutaneous pockets of pus involving several hair follicles.

Carcinoma Malignant neoplasm; cancer.

Carpopedal Spasm Abnormal flexion of the fingers and thumb, giving a clawlike appearance to the hands. It is often caused by severe hyperventilation.

Cataract Opacity in the lens of the eye.

Caudad Toward the tail.

Caustic Corrosive, capable of chemically destroying tissue.

Cellulitis Localized inflammation of soft tissue.

Centi Prefix denoting 1/100.

Central Nervous System (CNS) The brain and spinal cord.

Cephalad Craniad; towards the head.

Cerumen Modified sebum produced by glands in the skin of the external ear. Ear wax.

Cervix Neck. Often used to refer to the neck of the uterus where the vagina and the uterus are joined.

Chancre Hard, painless ulcer. Primary lesion of syphilis.

Cholecystectomy Surgical removal of the gall-bladder.

Cholecystitis Inflammation of the gall-bladder

Chondral Cartilaginous.

Chronic Pertaining to a disease with slow progression and long duration.

Clinical Death Cessation of respiration and heartbeat. It is reversible.

Clonic Alternating contraction and relaxation of muscles.

Coagulation Process of clot formation.

Cognitive Possessing normal ability to reason.

Coma Level of unconsciousness from which

the individual cannot be aroused regardless of the stimulus.

Comedo Blocked sebaceous duct characterized by black colored, oxidized sebum at opening to surface of skin; blackhead.

Concave Possessing a depressed or hollowed out surface.

Congenital Present at birth.

Conjunctiva The membrane that lines the eyelids and covers the surface of the eye which is exposed when the eyelids are retracted.

Constrict To make smaller.

Contusion Soft tissue injury, usually manifested by a bruise.

Convex Possessing an outwardly curved surface.

Cornea Transparent tissue covering the pupil of the eye.

Costal Pertaining to ribs.

Cravat Triangular bandage.

Crepitus Grating felt and heard when two roughened surfaces are rubbed together.

Crowning The appearance of the fetus at the vaginal orifice.

Cyanosis Bluish colored mucosa or skin resulting from hypoxia.

Cyst A fluid filled sac.

D

Debridement Surgical removal of dead tissue from a wound.

Decerebrate Posture Pathological position characterized by extension of the legs, and internal rotation and extension of the arms.

Decompression Sickness A syndrome produced when a rapid decrease in ambient pressure allows nitrogen dissolved in body tissue (blood, fat, muscle, etc.) to return to its gaseous state. Also known as "Caisson disease" or "The Bends."

Decontaminate To remove harmful foreign material from the body.

Decorticate Posture Pathological position characterized by extension of the legs and flexion of the arms at the elbows.

Decubitus Ulcer Ulceration caused by continuous pressure on one specific body area.

Deep Remote from the surface. Opposite of superficial.

Degenerative A process characterized by deterioration of tissue from its normal condition.

Dehydrate Remove or lose excessive amounts of fluids from the body.

Dehydration   Act of dehydrating or condition of being dehydrated.

Delirium Tremens   An archaic term used to describe alcohol withdrawal delirium. A condition characterized by visual, auditory and tactile hallucinations, incoherence, autonomic hyperactivity and tremulousness (tremors) caused by the abrupt withdrawal (discontinuance or decrease in the amount ingested) from alcohol. Also known as "DTs."

Delusion   A belief that has no basis in fact.

Dentalgia   Toothache.

Depressant   A substance which decreases the level of function of a patient. A sedative.

Depressed Skull Fracture   A skull fracture in which the bone fragments are displaced inwardly.

Depression   An abnormal mental state characterized by guilt over insignificant things, change in appetite, insomnia, lack of interest, lack of energy, decreased activity, inability to concentrate and thoughts of suicide.

Dermatitis   Inflammation of the skin.

Dermis   Inner layer of skin. The layer containing the sweat glands, neurovascular structures and hair follicles.

Diabetic Coma   State of unconsciousness caused by an inadequate supply of active insulin.

Diaphoresis   Excessive perspiration.

Diaphysis   Shaft portion of a long bone.

Diarrhea   Frequent voiding of watery stools.

Diffuse   General, non-localized.

Dilation   The act of expanding or enlarging circumferentially.

Diplopia   Double vision.

Dislocation   Condition which exists when a bone has been displaced from its joint.

Distal   Away from a point of reference, generally the heart.

Distended   Abnormally inflated or enlarged.

Diuretic   A substance which increases excretion of fluid by the kidneys.

Dorsal   Pertaining to the back.

Dressing   Protective covering applied directly to a wound.

Dysfunction   Abnormal function.

Dyskinesia   Difficulty performing movement.

Dysmenorrhea   Difficult, painful menstruation.

Dyspareunia   Painful sexual intercourse.

Dyspepsia   Indigestion.

Dysphagia Difficulty swallowing.

Dysphasia Inability to combine words to produce meaningful speech.

Dysphonia Difficulty speaking.

Dyspnea Complaining of "shortness of breath" or difficulty breathing.

Dysuria Painful, burning or difficult urination.

E

Ecchymosis Purplish discoloration caused by blood under the skin. A bruise.

Eclampsia A toxic condition of pregnancy associated with hypertension, edema, and seizures.

Ectopic Abnormal location.

Ectopic Pregnancy A pregnancy in which the fetus is implanted other than in the uterus.

Edema Local or generalized swelling.

Effusion The movement of fluid from tissues into a space; joint effusion, pleural effusion.

Electrocution Death caused by passage of electrical current through the body.

Embolism The sudden blocking of an artery or vein by a clot or foreign material.

Embolus   Any foreign matter carried in the bloodstream.

Emesis   Vomiting.

Emphysema   A chronic lung disease. Also the accumulation of air in tissues such as in subcutaneous emphysema.

Empyema   Pus in a body cavity, such as the thorax.

Encopresis   Uncontrollable defecation.

Endocrine   Internally secreting.

Endotracheal   Within the trachea.

Enophthalmos   A condition in which the eyeballs seem to be sunken deeply into their orbits.

Enteritis   Inflammation of the intestine.

Enucleate   To remove an eye from its orbit.

Enzyme   A protein catalyst.

Epidermis   The outermost, nonvascular layer of the skin.

Epidural   Located outside the outermost membrane that covers the brain or spinal cord.

Epigastric Region   The upper middle region of the abdomen.

Epiglottis   The cartilaginous flaplike structure superior to the larynx that prevents food from entering the trachea.

Epiglottitis A bacterial infection of the epiglottis.

Epilepsy A chronic neurological disorder marked by alteration of consciousness, abnormal motor behavior and sensory disturbances.

Epiphysis Distal to the physis, or growth plate.

Equilibrium Balance.

Eschar Thick crust that forms over burned tissue.

Esophagus That portion of the digestive tract between the pharynx and the stomach.

Estrogen One of the female sex hormones.

Etiology The cause of a medical problem.

Eustachian The tube from the middle ear to the throat. The auditory canal.

Evert To turn outward; to pronate.

Evisceration The penetration of the skin by abdominal organs.

Exacerbate To worsen a problem.

Expectorate Cough up.

Exsanguinate To bleed to death. To remove all the blood from a limb or body.

Extension The movement of a limb toward a straight condition.

External Pertaining to the outside.

External Auditory Canal The passage from the outer ear to the tympanic membrane.

External Ear The ear external to the tympanic membrane.

Extravasation Penetration of intravenous fluid out of a vein and into surrounding tissues.

Extremity An arm or leg.

Exudate A seepage of material, often pus, out of mucosal tissue.

F

Fainting A temporary, self resolving loss of consciousness. Psychogenic; syncope.

Fallopian Tubes The tubes from the ovaries to the uterus.

Fascia Fibrous tissue surrounding muscle, bone, or organs.

Fatigue Fracture A fracture resulting from repeated stress.

Febrile Pertaining to fever.

Femur The thigh bone.

Fetal Pertaining to the fetus.

Fetus   The unborn offspring.

Fibrin   Protein material used in blood clot formation.

Fibula   The smaller of the two bones of the lower leg.

Fistula   Abnormal opening between organs or from an organ to the skin.

Flaccid   Limp. Without muscular tone.

Flail Chest   The separation of the ribs from the sternum producing a freely moving segment of the rib cage.

Flashback   The appearance of blood in an intravenous catheter during venipuncture indicating entry into the vessel's lumen.

Flexion   Bending at a joint.

Follicle   A canal through the skin containing hair.

Fontanelles   The space between the bones of the skull of infants.

Foramen   A natural opening through a body structure.

Fossa   A depression below the level of the surrounding tissue.

Formed Elements   Red and white blood cells and platelets.

Frontal Forehead region of the head.

Frost Nip Superficial tissue freezing.

Frostbite Full thickness freezing of tissue.

Fulminant Developing very rapidly.

G

Gait The way a patient walks.

Gangrene Tissue death from inadequate blood supply.

Gastric Pertaining to the stomach.

Gastroenteritis Inflammation of the stomach and intestines.

Genital Pertaining to the reproductive organs.

Genu Pertaining to the knee.

Genu Recurvatum Back kneed.

Genu Valgum Knock kneed.

Genu Varum Bow legged.

Geriatric Pertaining to the elderly.

Gestation The period of fetal development.

Gingiva The gums. Soft tissue surrounding teeth.

Glaucoma A disorder characterized by increased pressure in the eyeball.

Glottis The true vocal cords and the opening between them.

Glucosuria Excretion of glucose in the urine.

Goiter Chronic, non-neoplastic enlargement of the thyroid gland.

Gonad Reproductive gland.

Goniometer Instrument used to measure angles to determine the range of motion of a joint.

Gout A disorder caused by excess uric acid in the body characterized by painful joints, usually the big toe.

Grand Mal Epileptic seizure characterized by generalized convulsions.

Gravid Pregnant.

Grippe Archaic lay term for influenza.

Guaiac A reagent which turns blue in the presence of iron. Used to check for the presence of occult blood in body fluids and excrement.

Guarding Protective, withdrawing reaction to palpation of a patient with abdominal pain.

Gynecomastia Excessive development of the male breast.

H

Hallucination   Sensory perception not based on reality.

Hallucinogen   An agent capable of stimulating hallucinations.

Hallux   The great toe.

Hematemesis   Vomiting blood.

Hematoma   A collection of blood in tissue; a blood clot.

Hematuria   Blood in the urine.

Hemiplegia   Paralysis of one side of the body.

Hemolysis   Abnormal disintegration of red blood cells.

Hemophilia   A hereditary blood disorder that interferes with coagulation.

Hemoptysis   Coughing up blood (from the lungs).

Hemorrhage   Excessive bleeding.

Hemostasis   To stop bleeding.

Hemothorax   Blood in the chest cavity.

Hepatitis   Inflammation of the liver.

Hepato   Pertaining to the liver.

Hepatomegaly   Enlargement of the liver.

Hepatotoxic   A substance possessing the potential to damage liver tissue.

Hernia Protrusion of an organ or organ part through the tissue that normally surrounds it.

Hirsutism Excessive body and/or facial hair.

Hives Raised patches on the skin characteristic of allergic reactions. Urticaria.

Homeostasis Maintenance of internal stability of a body.

Hormone Any one of the biochemical mediators produced by glands within the body.

Humerus The bone of the upper arm.

Hydrocele The collection of serous fluid within a sac. Usually used in reference to the scrotum.

Hypercarbia Excessive carbon dioxide in the body.

Hyperextension Overextension of a body part.

Hyperglycemia Increased concentration of glucose in the blood.

Hyperpnea Increased depth of respiration.

Hyperthermia Abnormally high body temperature.

Hypertrophy Increase in size of a body or organ part.

Hyperventilation Abnormally increased rate and depth of breathing.

Hyphema Blood in the anterior chamber of the eye.

Hypocarbia Abnormally low carbon dioxide in the blood.

Hypoglottus Undersurface of the tongue.

Hypoglycemia An abnormally low concentration of glucose in the blood.

Hyponatremia Abnormally low sodium in the blood.

Hypopharynx The distal portion of the pharynx.

Hypothermia Abnormally low body temperature.

Hypoventilation Reduced rate and depth of breathing.

Hypovolemia Abnormally low amount of blood and fluids in the body.

Hypoxemia Inadequate oxygen in the blood.

Hypoxia Inadequate oxygenation at the cell level.

Hysterectomy Surgical removal of the uterus.

I

Icterus Jaundice: yellow discoloration of skin and conjunctiva caused by bile pigment.

Idiopathic   Of unknown origin.

Ileum   The portion of the small intestine from the jejunum to the cecum.

Iliac   Superior portion of the hip bone.

Ilium   The broad, uppermost portions of the hip bone.

Imbricated   Overlapped, like scales or roof shingles.

Impaction   Firmly packed.

Impaled Object   An object embedded in the wound it has produced.

Impetigo   Bacterial skin infection characterized by crusted, weeping lesions.

Impotent   Unable to achieve an erection.

Incipient   Early.

Incision   A wound with smooth edges.

Incontinence   Inability to prevent voiding.

Incus   The middle bone of the middle ear.

Indwelling Catheter   A plastic tube designed to remain within the lumen of a tube.

Infarction   Localized tissue death due to the interruption of its supply of oxygenated blood.

Infectious   Capable of causing infection.

Inferior   Toward the feet.

Ingestion   Taking a substance through the mouth.

Inguinal   Pertaining to the groin.

Insomnia   Inability to sleep.

Insulin Shock   Severe hypoglycemia.

Inotropic   A drug that increases the force of cardiac contractions.

Integument   The skin.

Intercostal   Between the ribs.

Intermammary   The imaginary horizontal line that connects the nipples.

Internal   Deep; away from the surface.

Inversion   Turning inward. Supination.

Ipecac, Syrup of   An emetic.

IPPB   Intermittent positive pressure breathing device.

Ipsilateral   On the same side.

Iris   Colored portion of the eye that surrounds the pupil.

Ischemia   Tissue damage due to decreased oxygen.

Ischium   The lowermost portion of the hip bone.

Islets of Langerhans   The cells in the pancreas that produce insulin.

Isotonic   Having the same osmotic pressure as intracellular fluid.

IV   Intravenous.

J

Jaundice Excessive bile pigments in the bloodstream which produce a yellow discoloration of the skin and conjunctiva.

Joint Articulation of adjacent bones.

Joint Capsule Fibrous sac that encloses a joint.

Jugular Notch Superior aspect of the sternum.

Jugular Venous Distention Engorgement of the jugular veins.

Junctional Rhythm A dysrhythmia originating in the atrioventricular junction.

K

Ketoacidosis The condition which occurs when circulating insulin is inadequate. Fat is metabolized to ketones and acids. The cause of diabetic coma.

Ketonuria Presence of ketones in the urine.

Kussmaul's Respirations Deep, rapid breathing caused by the body's attempt to counteract acidosis.

L

Labia The folds of skins and mucous membranes that comprise the vulva.

Labor Contraction of the uterus to expel the fetus.

Laceration Tearing or cutting of body tissue.

Lacrimal Gland Tear gland.

Lactation Secretion of milk.

Laparotomy Incision into the abdominal cavity.

Laryngeal Pertaining to the larynx.

Laryngectomee Person who has had a laryngectomy.

Laryngectomy Surgical removal of the larynx.

Laryngospasm Spastic constriction of the larynx.

Larynx Voice box.

Lateral Toward the side. Away from midline.

Lateral Recumbent Lying on the side.

Lateral Rotation Turning of the foot or hand away from the midline.

Lavage To wash out a body part, such as an eye, stomach, etc.

Lethargy Lack of activity.

Leukemia Abnormal proliferation of white blood cells (leukocytes).

Leukorrhea Yellowish white, thick vaginal discharge.

Libido Sexual desire.

Ligament Fibrous tissues which connect bone to bone.

Ligate To tie off a tube or blood vessel.

Lipoma A benign tumor composed of fat cells.

Litigation Lawsuit.

Livid Having a dark blue skin color.

Localized Confined to a small area.

Lordosis Concavity of the spine, such as is normal in the lumbar region.

Lower Extremity The legs and feet.

Lucid Having clear meaning. Without confusion.

Lumbar Lower back (vertebrae) between the ribs and pelvis.

Lumen The channel through a tube such as a vein.

Lumpectomy Surgical removal of a mass (or lump) from the breast with little disruption of surrounding tissue.

Lupus *See* Systemic Lupus Erythematosus.

Lymphangitis Inflammation of the lymphatic vessels resulting in a discernible red streak that appears to move proximally from the site of infection that initially caused the inflammation.

Lymph Node Any one of the bodies located along the lymphatic vessels that act as filters for the lymphatic system.

Lymphoma Malignant tumor(s) of the lymphatic system or any of its components.

M

Macerate Soften by soaking or keeping wet.

Malaise Generalized feeling of discomfort.

Malignancy A disorder that is life-threatening and difficult to manage.

Malleolus The bony protuberance on each side of the ankle.

Malleus One of the three bones of the middle ear.

Malunion Improper or incomplete healing of a fracture.

Mandible Lower jawbone.

Manubrium The upper portion of the sternum above the angle of Louis.

Masticate   To chew.

Mastoid   The portion of the skull that lies immediately posterior to the ear.

Maxilla   Upper jawbone.

Meconium   First discharge of intestinal material from a newborn.

Medial   Toward the midline of the body.

Mediastinal Region (Mediastinum)   The space within the thorax between the left and right pleural spaces.

Medulla   The portion of the brain that controls vegetative functions.

Melanin   Skin pigment.

Meninges   The membranes covering the brain and spinal cord.

Meningitis   Inflammation of the meninges.

Menopause   The permanent cessation of menstrual activity.

Menorrhagia   Excessive flow during menstruation.

Menses   The discharge that occurs during menstruation.

Menstruation   Sloughing off of the uterine lining each month by a woman of childbearing age.

Metacarpal   The bones of the hand from the wrist to the fingers.

Metastasis The spreading of a disease from one part of the body to another.

Metatarsal The bones of the foot extending from the ankles to the toes.

Midclavicular Line The vertical line beginning in the middle of the clavicle and running inferiorly and parallel to the midline.

Midline The vertical line down the center of the body dividing it into right and left halves.

Miosis Pupillary constriction.

Miscarriage Spontaneous abortion.

Mitral Valve The valve between the left atrium and left ventricle.

Morbidity Illness.

Morbilliform Having the appearance of measles.

Mortality Death.

Mnemonic Series of words to assist memorization.

Mucosa Mucous membrane; mucous producing tissue.

Mucous Membrane A membrane that lines many organs of the body and contains mucous-secreting glands.

Multifocal Arising from, or pertaining to, many foci or locations.

Multipara   A woman who has had more than two pregnancies; also called "multip."

Myalgia   Muscle pain or aches.

Mydriasis   Pupillary dilatation.

Myocardium   Heart muscle.

Myoclonus   Rhythmic spasms of muscle.

N

Narcolepsy   Periods of sleep occurring suddenly and at unusual times.

Nasopharyngeal   Pertaining to the nasopharynx.

Nasopharynx   The pharynx above the palate.

Nausea   Having the urge to vomit.

Necrosis   Tissue death.

Necrotic   Pertaining to dead tissue.

Neonatal Period   The first month of life beginning immediately at birth.

Neonate   A newborn.

Neoplasm   A mass of tissue exhibiting unusually rapid growth. A tumor.

Neoplastic   Pertaining to a neoplasm.

Nephrotoxic   A substance that causes damage to kidney tissue.

Neuralgia Pain along the distribution of a nerve.

Neurotoxic Poisonous to nerve tissue.

Nocturia The necessity to get up at night to urinate.

Nocturnal Pertaining to nighttime.

Nonviable Unable to sustain life without extraordinary assistance.

Nosocomial Infection Hospital acquired disease.

Nulligravida A woman who has never been pregnant.

Nullpara A woman who has never borne a child.

Nummular Coin shaped.

Nystagmus Rapid oscillation of the eyes.

O

Obese Grossly overweight.

Oblique Deviating from perpendicular.

Occipital Pertaining to the back of the skull.

Occiput The back of the skull.

Occlude To close off; obstruct.

Occult Not obvious or easily recognizable.

Ocular Pertaining to the eye.

Olecranon Process The tip of the elbow.

Oliguria Abnormally low urine output.

Oncology The study of neoplasms.

Opisthotonos A convulsive, rigid arching of the back.

Oral Pertaining to the mouth.

Orbits The cavities in the skull that hold the eyeballs.

Oropharynx Area between the soft palate and the epiglottis.

Orthopnea Difficulty breathing when lying down.

Orthostatic Decrease in blood pressure upon sitting or standing.

Ossicle One of the three bones of the middle ear.

Osteoporosis Abnormally increased porosity of bone.

Ototoxic A substance which has a poisonous effect on the ear, usually by chemically damaging the associated nerves.

Ovulation Release of a mature ovum from the ovaries.

Ovum Egg.

P

Palate Roof of the mouth.

Palatine Pertaining to the roof of the mouth.

Palliative Easing the symptoms of a disease without curing the underlying problem.

Pallor Paleness.

Palmar Pertaining to the palm of the hand.

Palpate To examine by feeling with the hand.

Palpation The act of feeling with the hand.

Palpitation Forceful heartbeat that is perceived by the patient as a "pounding heart."

Pancreatitis Inflammation of the pancreas.

Paradoxical Movement Motion opposite to normal movement.

Paralysis Loss of motor function.

Paraplegia The loss of sensation and motion in the lower extremities.

Parenchyma The substance of an organ.

Parenteral The administration of a medication by injection.

Paresis Weakness.

Paresthesia Pins-and-needles sensation.

Parietal Bones The bones that form the roof and sides of the skull.

Patella   The kneecap.

Patency   The state of being intact.

Patent   Intact.

Pectoriloquy   The transmission of voice by thickened secretions within the lungs, so that it can be clearly heard on auscultation.

Pedal   Pertaining to the foot.

Pelvic Cavity   The lowermost portion of the abdominal cavity.

Pelvis   Hip bone.

Percussion   The tapping of the body to determine the density of the underlying structures based upon the resulting sound.

Percutaneous   Through the skin.

Perfusion   Adequacy of blood supply.

Pericardial Effusion   Excess fluid within the pericardium.

Pericardium (Pericardial Sac)   The sac surrounding the heart.

Perineum   The area between the genitals and the anus.

Periorbital   Around the eyes.

Periosteum   The fibrous tissue covering bone.

Peristalsis (Peristaltic Wave)   Waves of muscular contraction.

Peritoneum   The membrane lining the abdominal cavity.

Peritonitis   Inflammation of the peritoneum.

Petechiae   Pinpoint hemorrhages under the skin.

Petit Mal Seizure   Seizure activity characterized by a momentary loss of awareness without convulsions.

Phalanx (pl. Phalanges)   Bone of the finger or toe.

Phantom Pain   Pain actually experienced by an amputee that he perceives as originating in the amputated limb.

Phlebitis   Inflammation of a vein.

Phlegm   Archaic term used to describe expectorated mucus.

Phobia   An abnormal fear of some specific thing.

Photophobia   Painful hypersensitivity to light.

Pica   Appetite for substances not normally considered food.

Pinna   The external ear.

Plantar   Pertaining to the sole of the foot.

Plasma   The fluid portion of blood without red or white cells.

Platelet An element in the blood that is necessary for blood clotting.

Pleura Membrane that lines the outer surfaces of the lungs and the inner surface of the thoracic cavity.

Pleuritis Inflammation of the pleura; pleurisy.

Pneumonectomy Surgical removal of a lung.

Pneumothorax Free air in the pleural cavity.

Polydactyly Presence of more than five fingers or toes on one hand or foot.

Polydipsia Excessive thirst or intake of fluids.

Polyp A mass of tissue attached to the surface of some other tissue by a pedicle or stalk.

Polyphagia Excessive eating.

Polyuria Excessive urination.

Popliteal Fossa The posterior aspect of the knee joint.

Posterior Toward the back or behind.

Postictal The period of time immediately following an epileptic seizure.

Postpartum After delivery.

Post Prandial Following a meal.

Prandial Pertaining to a meal.

Precocious Indicating early development or maturity.

Prenatal Before birth.

Prepubescent Before puberty; childhood.

Priapism Persistent abnormal erection of the penis.

Primipara The first pregnancy.

Progeria A disorder characterized by extremely accelerated aging.

Progesterone Ovarian hormone.

Prognosis Probable outcome.

Prolapsed Cord A delivery in which the umbilical cord presents before the infant's body.

Pronation Turning the hand palm down; eversion.

Prone Lying face down.

Proptosis The appearance of an eyeball bulging out of its orbit.

Prostate A gland at the base of the male urinary bladder.

Prosthesis Artificial part.

Prostration Collapse.

Protocol Preestablished plan for the management of a specific medical problem.

Proximal Closer to a point of reference.

Pruritus Itching.

Ptarmus Sneezing.

Ptosis Falling down of the upper eyelid into a semiclosed position; drooping.

Puberty The period of time during which a child develops into an adult.

Pulmonary Pertaining to the lungs.

Pulsatile Throbbing rhythmically, as with the heartbeat.

Purulent Containing pus: foul smelling.

Pus Semisolid matter produced by infection.

Pyogenic Producing pus.

Pyrexia Fever.

Pyrogenic Causing fever.

Pyrosis Substernal discomfort of a burning nature; heartburn.

Pyuria Pus in the urine.

Q

Quadrant One quarter of an area.

Quadriplegia Paralysis of arms and legs.

Querulent One who is distrustful, quarrelsome, difficult to satisfy, quick to anger.

Quickening Movement of the fetus in utero felt by the mother.

R

Raccoon Sign (Coon's eyes) Bilateral, periorbital ecchymoses sometimes seen with skull fractures.

Radius The bone on the thumb side of the lower arm.

Rales Crackles; adventitious breath sounds heard as air moves through congested bronchioles. Sounds similar to strands of hair being rubbed together.

Rectum The distal portion of the digestive tract.

Recumbent Lying horizontally.

Reduce To restore a fractured or dislocated part to its normal position.

Referred Pain Pain felt at a location other than where it originates.

Reflex Involuntary contraction of a muscle by applying an external, mechanical stimulus to the muscle or its tendon.

Reflux Flow opposite the normal direction.

Regimen Pattern of living, incorporating diet, drugs, exercise, sleep, etc.

Regurgitation The passive flow of gastric contents into the pharynx from the stomach.

Renal   Pertaining to the kidney.

Respiration   The exchange of oxygen and carbon dioxide between the lungs, blood, and tissues.

Resuscitation   The effort to manually restore normal heart and/or lung functions.

Retina   The tissue in the back of the eye that converts visual images to nerve impulses.

Retractions   The use of accessory muscles for ventilation.

Rhonchi   Lung sounds, sometimes referred to as musical, usually caused by secretions in the lower airways.

Rhinitis   Inflammation of the nasal mucosa.

Rhinoplasty   Surgical repair of a defect in nasal structure.

Rigor Mortis   Stiffness of death.

Rotator Cuff   The group of four muscles: the supraspinatus, infraspinatus, teres minor and subscapularis that surround and mobilize the shoulder joint.

S

Sacral   Pertaining to the sacrum.

Sacrum   The last five vertebrae.

Saline A solution of sodium chloride.

Scald Burn caused by hot liquid or steam.

Scapula Shoulder blade.

Sclera The hard outer layer of the eyeball. The "white" of the eye.

Sclerosis Term used to describe hardening of a normally soft tissue.

Scoliosis Lateral curvature of the spine.

Scotoma Blind spot in the patient's visual field.

Scrotal Pertaining to the scrotum.

Sebum Material secreted by sebaceous glands.

Sepsis Presence of infectious organisms in the body.

Septum A dividing wall of tissue.

Sequela Problems that follow and are caused by a disease or disorder.

Serum The liquid portion of blood with the fibrin and cells removed.

Shock Inadequate tissue perfusion.

Sign Objective findings.

Sinus A cavernous opening in bone.

Soft Palate The muscular tissue at the superior posterior aspect of the mouth.

Spasm A sudden involuntary muscle contraction.

Sphygmomanometer   Blood pressure cuff.

Splenomegaly   Enlarged spleen.

Sprain   Injury to the ligaments surrounding a joint.

Sputum   Expectorated material.

Stapes   One of the three bones of the middle ear.

Stasis   The slowing down or cessation of the flow of body fluid. Usually refers to blood, urine, etc.

Stat   An abbreviation meaning "immediately."

Steatorrhea   The passage of large amounts of undigested fat in the feces.

Stenosis   Narrowing or stricture of a vessel.

Status Asthmaticus   Severe asthmatic episode which is unresponsive to medication.

Status Epilepticus   The occurrence of continuous seizure activity.

Sternal   Pertaining to the sternum.

Sternum   The breast bone.

Stertorous   Snoring respirations.

Stoma   A small artificial opening.

Strain   Injury caused by the stretching of the muscle beyond its natural limits.

Stricture Abnormal narrowing of a duct or vessel.

Stridor High-pitched sound associated with upper airway obstruction.

Stroke Cerebrovascular accident; CVA

Stupor Reduced level of consciousness; confusion.

Subcutaneous Beneath the skin.

Subluxation Incomplete dislocation of a joint. One in which the bone ends remain in some contact.

Substernal Deep to the sternum.

Superficial Near the surface.

Superior Above another body part.

Supernumerary An extra body part such as supernumerary nipples, etc.

Supination Turning the arm so that the palm faces upward, or inversion of the foot.

Supine Lying face-upward.

Suprapubic Lower central abdominal region above the pubis.

Symptom Subjective complaint of a medical problem.

Syncope Fainting; brief, self-resolving loss of consciousness.

Syndactyly The condition of having webbed digits.

Syndrome A collection of signs and symptoms peculiar to a disorder or disease process.

Synovial Fluid The fluid that lubricates joints.

Systemic Affecting the body as a whole.

Systemic Lupus Erythematosus An autoimmune inflammatory process involving multiple organ systems. Etiology is unknown.

T

Tachycardia Abnormally rapid heart rate.

Tachypnea Abnormally rapid respiration.

Tactile Pertaining to the sense of touch.

Tactile Fremitus Vibration palpated on the patient's chest while he is speaking.

Tarsal Pertaining to the ankle.

Telangiectasia Dilation of the capillaries just under the skin surface resulting in the appearance of purplish spider webs.

Temporal The side of the head above the ears.

Tendon Fibrous connective tissue that attaches muscles to bone.

Testicular Torsion Twisting of the testicle within the scrotum.

Tetralogy A group of four signs, symptoms, etc. that have something in common.

Thenar Eminence The mass of tissue at the base of the thumb.

Thoracic Pertaining to the chest.

Thorax The cavity between the neck and the diaphragm.

Thrombus A clot formed inside a blood vessel.

Thrush Oral infection by the Candida albicans fungus.

Tibia The shin bone. The larger bone in the lower leg.

Tic The spasmodic twitching of a facial muscle.

Tinnitus Abnormal ringing in the ears.

Tonic Persistent contraction.

Topical On the surface.

Torticollis A condition caused by contraction of the muscles on one side of the neck resulting in the head being pulled to that side, while the face points to the opposite side.

Trachea Windpipe.

Transillumination The examination of a body region by passing light through it.

Transverse From side to side.

Trauma Injury.

Tragus The cartilaginous projection anterior to the external auditory canal.

Trendelenburg Position Supine with legs raised and head lowered; "shock position."

Tricuspid The valve between the right atrium and right ventricle.

Trimester One-third of a pregnancy.

Trismus A spasm of the jaw muscles causing the teeth to remain clenched tightly shut.

Turgor Fullness of the subcutaneous tissue.

Tympanic Membrane The eardrum.

U

Ulcer An open lesion.

Ulna The larger bone of the lower arm.

Umbilicus "Belly button."

Upper Extremity The shoulder girdle, arm and hand.

Ureter The tubes that convey urine from the kidneys to the bladder.

Urethra The tube that carries urine from the bladder to the urethral orifice.

Urgency Overwhelming desire to void.

Urticaria Hives; generalized, pruritic, raised wheals.

Uvula The small growth of soft tissue hanging from the soft palate.

Uterus The organ that holds and nourishes the fetus.

V

Vagina The canal from the uterus to the vulva.

Vallecula The slot at the base of the tongue and posterior to the epiglottis.

Vascular Pertaining to blood vessels.

Vasoconstriction Narrowing of the diameter of a blood vessel.

Vasodilation Increasing the diameter of blood vessels.

Vein Any blood vessel that returns blood to the heart.

Venous   Pertaining to a vein.

Ventral   Pertaining to the abdomen or anterior aspect of the body.

Venule   A small vein.

Vernix   The cheesy material found on newborns.

Verruca   General term for wart (pl. Verrucae).

Vertebrae   The bones of the spinal column.

Vertigo   The sensation that the surrounding area is spinning around the patient.

Viable   Capable of living or being kept alive.

Virulence   The ability of a pathogen to provoke a disease process in a host.

Void   To excrete waste products; release urine or feces.

Vomiting   The active expulsion of gastric contents through the mouth; emesis.

Vomitus   The material ejected from the stomach by vomiting.

W

Wheal   Area of skin raised by subcutaneous fluid.

Wheeze   A high pitched, whistling sound characterizing obstruction or spasm of the lower airways.

Word Salad   The jumble of meaningless words or phrases spoken by an individual afflicted with certain mental disorders.

X

Xiphoid Process   The knifelike protrusion at the inferior edge of the sternum.

Z

Zygoma   The bone forming the inferiolateral aspect of the orbit, as well as that portion of the floor of the orbit.

Adult Glasgow Coma Scale

EYE OPENING:

None	1
To Pain Stimulus	2
To Verbal Stimulus	3
Spontaneous	4

BEST VERBAL RESPONSE:

None	1
Incomprehensible Sounds	2
Inappropriate Words	3

| Confused | 4 |
| Oriented | 5 |

BEST MOTOR RESPONSE:

None	1
Abnormal Extension (Decerebrate)	2
Abnormal Flexion (Decorticate)	3
Withdraws From Pain	4
Localizes Pain	5
Obeys Commands	6

Pediatric Glasgow Coma Scale

Eye Opening

> 1 year old	< 1 year old	
None	None	1
To Pain	To Pain	2
To Verbal Stimulus	To Shout	3
Spontaneously	Spontaneously	4

Best Verbal Response

> 5 year old	2 − 5 year old	0 − 23 months	
None	None	None	1
Incomprehensible Sounds	Grunts	Grunts, Restless	2
Inappropriate Words	Cries and/or Screams	Inappropriate Crying and/or Screaming	3
Disoriented but Converses	Inappropriate Words	Cries, Consolable	4
Oriented and Converses	Appropriate Words and Phrases	Smiles, Coos, Cries When Appropriate	5

Best Motor Response

> 1 year old	< 1 year old	
None	None	1
Abn. Extension (Decerebrate)	Abn. Extension (Decerebrate)	2
Abn. Flexion (Decorticate)	Abn. Flexion	3
Flexion To Painful Stimulus	Normal Flexion	4
Localizes Pain (pushes stimulus away)	Localizes Pain (moves away from stimulus)	5
Obeys Commands	Spontaneous	6

112

Trauma Score

GLASGOW COMA SCORE

14–15	5
11–13	4
8–10	3
5–9	2
3–4	1

RESPIRATORY RATE

10–24 / minute	4
25–35 / minute	3
> 35 / minute	2
1–9 / minute	1
0 / minute	0

RESPIRATORY EFFORT

Normal	1
Retractive	0

SYSTOLIC BLOOD PRESSURE

> 89 mm Hg	4
70–89 mm Hg	3
50–69 mm Hg	2
0–49 mm Hg	1
0 mm Hg	0

CAPILLARY REFILL

< 3 seconds	2
> 2 seconds	1
None	0

TOTAL **0 – 16**

APGAR
Score

ACTIVITY

Limp	0
Some flexion	1
Active, much flexion	2

PULSE

None	0
< 100 / minute	1
> 100 / minute	2

GRIMACE REFLEX TO SUCTION

None	0
Some grimacing	1
Sneezes, coughs, or cries	2

COLOR

Blue or very pale	0
Pink body, blue hands/feet	1
Pink all over	2

RESPIRATIONS

None	0
Irregular, ineffective, bradypneic	1
Rhythmic, effective, crying	2

Muscle Strength Grading*

No contraction	0
Slight contraction	1
Full range of motion with assistance to overcome gravity	2
Full range of motion without assistance to overcome gravity	3
Full range of motion against light resistance	4
Full range of motion against heavy resistance	5

*Expressed as the appropriate value over 5 possible, i.e. "+5/5" is normal muscle strength.

AMSIT

MENTAL STATUS EXAMINATION

APPEARANCE

Physical appearance—age, sex, etc.

Attitude toward examiner—cooperative, sarcastic, etc.

Unusual activity—pacing, rocking, etc.

Evidence of emotion—wringing hands, wrinkled brow, gritted teeth, tears, etc.

Senseless repetitious acts—tics, gestures, etc.

Attention disorders—distractibility, detachment, etc.

Abnormalities in speech—slurred speech, inability to speak, etc.

MOOD

Type—elated, depressed, euthymic, etc.

Intensity of mood.

Swings from one extreme to other.

Appropriateness.

SENSORIUM

Level of consciousness—alert and oriented to time, person, place and purpose.

Memory—immediate, short term, long term.

Calculations—simple addition, subtraction, etc.

INTELLECT

Estimate current level of mental function—average, retarded, etc.

General knowledge—President, recent events.

Vocabulary—appropriate for age, education, environment.

THOUGHT

Form—logical, reasonable association, speed, etc.

Content—suicidal, homicidal, delusions, etc.

Judgement—sensible, appropriate, etc.

Abstracting abilities—explaining proverbs, etc.

Insight—patient's awareness of his psychological problems.

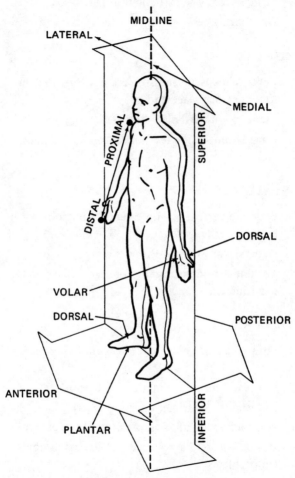

FIGURE 1. Anatomic Positions

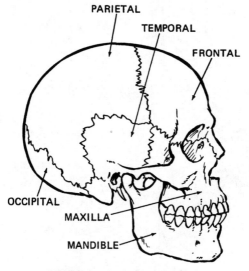

FIGURE 2. Regions of the Skull

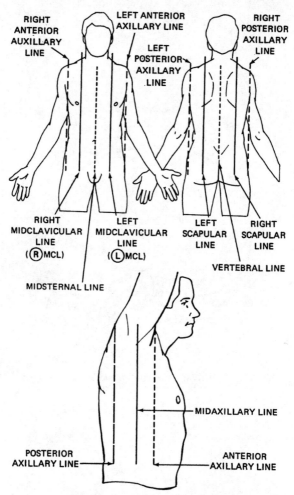

FIGURE 3. Thoracic Landmarks

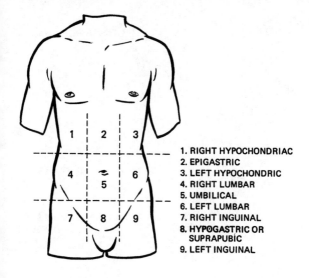

1. RIGHT HYPOCHONDRIAC
2. EPIGASTRIC
3. LEFT HYPOCHONDRIC
4. RIGHT LUMBAR
5. UMBILICAL
6. LEFT LUMBAR
7. RIGHT INGUINAL
8. HYPOGASTRIC OR SUPRAPUBIC
9. LEFT INGUINAL

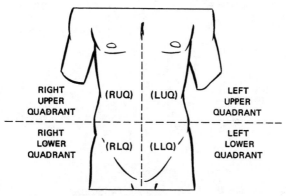

FIGURE 4. Abdominal Regions

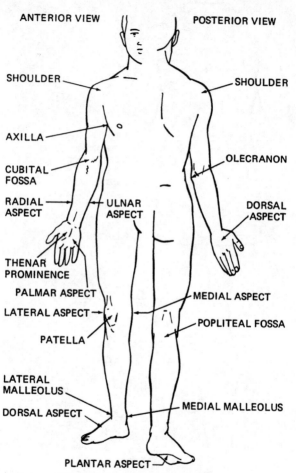

FIGURE 5. Areas of the Extremities

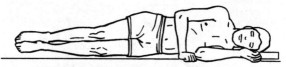

LEFT (SIDE DOWN) LATERALLY RECUMBENT
OR
LEFT (SIDE DOWN) LATERAL DECUBITUS

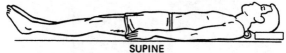

SUPINE

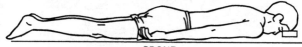

PRONE

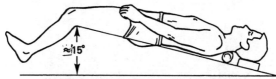

≈15°

TRENDELENBURG (OR SHOCK) POSITION

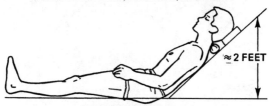

≈ 2 FEET

FOWLER'S POSITION

FIGURE 6. Body Positions

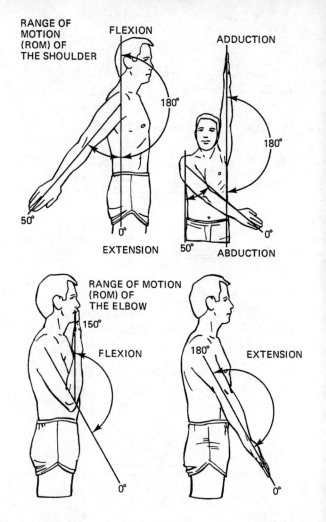

FIGURE 7. Range of Motion (ROM) of the Shoulder and the Elbow

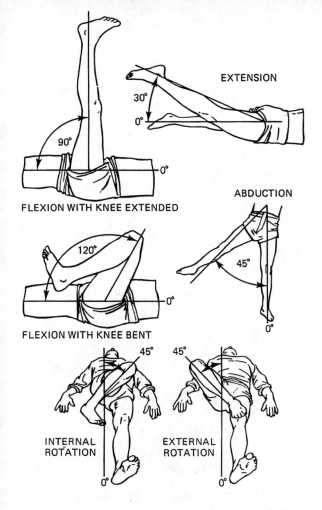

FIGURE 8. Range of Motion (ROM) of the Hip

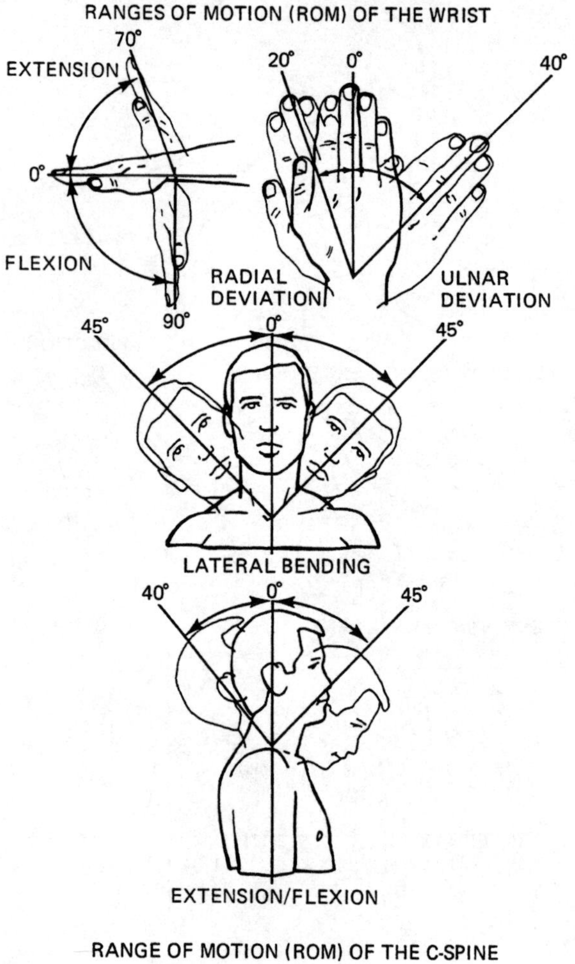

RANGES OF MOTION (ROM) OF THE WRIST

EXTENSION

70°

0°

FLEXION

90°

20°   0°

40°

RADIAL
DEVIATION

ULNAR
DEVIATION

45°   0°   45°

LATERAL BENDING

40°   0°   45°

EXTENSION/FLEXION

RANGE OF MOTION (ROM) OF THE C-SPINE

FIGURE 9. Range of Motion (ROM) of the Wrist and the C-Spine

RANGES OF MOTION (ROM) OF THE KNEE

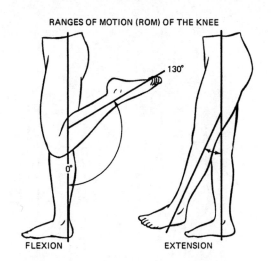

FLEXION   EXTENSION

RANGES OF MOTION (ROM) OF THE ANKLE

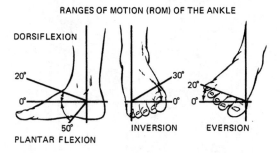

DORSIFLEXION

PLANTAR FLEXION

INVERSION   EVERSION

FIGURE 10. Range of Motion (ROM) of the Knee

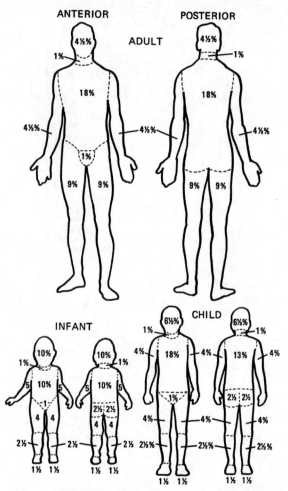

FIGURE 11. Percent of Surface Area

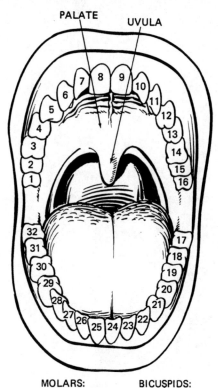

PALATE   UVULA

MOLARS:

1, 2, 3, 14, 15, 16,
17, 18, 19, 30, 31, 32

CUSPIDS:

6, 11, 22, 27

BICUSPIDS:

4, 5, 12, 13,
20, 21, 28, 29

INCISORS:

7, 8, 9, 10,
23, 24, 25, 26

FIGURE 12.   Dental Chart

131